Title: One Meal a Day (OMAD) Fasting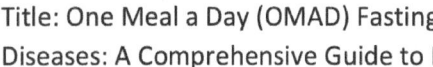
Diseases: A Comprehensive Guide to I

Table of Contents

1. Introducing OMAD - The Game-Changer for Chronic Pain and Autoimmune Warriors

- What is OMAD?
- How OMAD Works its Magic
- The Potential Benefits of OMAD

2. Understanding Chronic Pain and Autoimmune Diseases - The Real Struggles We Face

- Chronic Pain: The Invisible Battle
- Unraveling Autoimmune Diseases
- Navigating the Challenges of Autoimmunity

3. The Science Behind OMAD - How It's a Total Game-Changer

- OMAD and Metabolism
- Insulin and OMAD
- Energy Utilization on OMAD

4. Benefits of OMAD for Chronic Pain and Autoimmune Warriors - Get Ready to Be Amazed!

- Increased Energy Levels
- Enhanced Mental Clarity
- Potential Weight Management
- Managing Inflammation and Autoimmunity

5. Combining OMAD Fasting with Other Lifestyle Changes

- Exercise and Movement for Pain Relief

- Stress Management and Mindfulness
- Quality Sleep and Its Role in Healing

6. Troubleshooting and Overcoming Challenges

- Dealing with Plateaus
- Common Fasting Side Effects and How to Address Them

7. Crafting a Customized OMAD Meal Plan

- Navigating Nutritional Needs
- Building a Balanced OMAD Meal
- Embracing Variety and Culinary Creativity

8. Mindful Eating on OMAD - Savoring Every Bite

- The Power of Mindful Eating
- Avoiding Emotional Eating Traps
- Mindful Eating Tips for OMAD Success

9. The Social Aspect of OMAD - Navigating Family and Social Gatherings

- Creative Ways to Eat with Family and Friends
- Communicating Your OMAD Lifestyle
- Staying Committed Amidst Social Challenges

10. Celebrating Progress and Staying Motivated

- Recognizing Non-Scale Victories
- The Power of Progress Photos
- Creating a Supportive OMAD Community

Author Introduction

Hey there, amazing readers! I'm Jessica Cooper, a warrior with a passion for health, wellness, and embracing the power of One Meal a Day (OMAD). Life threw me some curveballs, and I found myself diagnosed with lupus at the age of 17, and later, multiple sclerosis at 32. These illnesses challenged me both physically and mentally, making it tough to lose weight due to medications and hospital stays that left me feeling weak.

But guess what? I'm not one to back down from a challenge! I dived headfirst into the world of OMAD, seeking ways to reclaim control over my health and well-being. It wasn't an easy journey - there were ups, downs, and repeat efforts to shed those extra pounds.

Through trials, errors, and countless learning experiences, I found my groove with OMAD. It became my lifeline, empowering me to manage my chronic conditions, improve my overall health, and feel like a true warrior in control of my destiny.

In this ebook, I'm thrilled to share my story and knowledge with you. We'll explore the wonders of OMAD, how it can benefit those facing chronic pain and autoimmune conditions, and how to embrace this lifestyle in the most rewarding way.

I want this book to be your go-to guide, your support system, and your source of inspiration. Together, we'll discover the true power of OMAD and how it can become a catalyst for transformative changes in your life. So, let's dive in, my fellow warriors, and unlock the incredible potential that lies ahead! 💪✨

Introduction

Living with chronic pain and autoimmune disorders can be frightening and intimidating. Conventional treatments frequently focus on symptom management; but, what if there was a natural strategy that might bring relief and possibly reverse the effects of these conditions? Fasting for one meal a day (OMAD) is a potential strategy that can improve lives by fostering healing from within.

In this ebook, we will explore the powerful effects of OMAD fasting on chronic pain and autoimmune diseases. We'll delve into the science behind fasting, its impact on the immune system, and how it can bring relief and enhance the body's self-healing abilities. Throughout the book, we will provide practical guidance, tips, and delicious recipes to help you incorporate OMAD fasting into your life and experience the benefits firsthand.

(disclaimer I am not a Doctor please consult with a professional before using any tips concerning omad and your disorder)

Chapter 1: Introducing OMAD - The Game-Changer for Chronic Pain and Autoimmune Warriors

Yo, what's up, fellow warriors? Welcome to the world of OMAD - One Meal a Day - where we're about to embark on a journey that'll transform how we deal with chronic pain and autoimmune conditions! So, buckle up, 'cause we're about to level up our health game!

In this chapter, we'll break down the basics of OMAD like we're spilling the tea at a party. We'll learn what OMAD is all about, how it works its magic on our bodies, and the potential benefits it brings to the table (or, uh, plate!). Get ready to embrace a lifestyle that's gonna empower us to take charge of our health like never before!

1. **OMAD Unmasked:** Ever heard of a superhero called OMAD? Get ready to meet the one-meal wonder that's about to flip the script on how you tackle chronic pain and those pesky autoimmune battles. Say

goodbye to confusion and hello to the ultimate OMAD 101 crash course!

2. **Magic in the Fasting Lane:** Imagine this – eating just one meal a day and watching your body transform like a boss. We're talking boosted metabolism, potential weight loss, and a whole lot of energy. Get ready to learn how OMAD does its enchanting dance with your body's internal workings.

3. **Benefits Galore, Baby:** Hold onto your hats, 'cause we're spilling the beans on the potential perks of rocking the OMAD lifestyle. From newfound energy levels to a potential immune system boost, OMAD ain't just about skipping meals – it's a full-blown wellness party you won't wanna miss. Let's get this OMAD party started, shall we?

Chapter 2: Understanding Chronic Pain and Autoimmune Diseases - The Real Struggles We Face

Alright, let's get real here. Chronic pain and autoimmune diseases can be a straight-up rollercoaster ride. It's like having an internal battle with our own bodies! We'll dive deep into the nitty-gritty of what these conditions are and how they mess with our lives. We'll talk about the struggles we face daily - the pain, the fatigue, and those dreaded flare-ups. But here's the thing - we're in this together, and we're gonna find ways to rise above these challenges like the fierce warriors we are!

> Chronic pain, it's like that uninvited guest who just won't leave, right? We all know pain, from the occasional headache to those persistent aches and pains that seem to have taken up permanent residence in our lives. But chronic pain is something different; it's the marathon runner of discomfort, constantly reminding us it's there. We'll delve into the science behind chronic pain, exploring how it disrupts our daily lives and makes even the simplest tasks feel like climbing Mount Everest.
>
> Now, let's talk about autoimmune diseases – the body's internal rebels. These conditions are like having a group of your own immune

cells turn against you, mistaking your healthy cells for invaders. It's confusing, frustrating, and often exhausting. Autoimmunity isn't a one-size-fits-all deal; it's a spectrum of disorders, from the well-known ones like rheumatoid arthritis and lupus to lesser-known warriors like Hashimoto's thyroiditis. We'll dig deep into the complexities, the mystery of flare-ups, and the unique challenges you face as someone navigating the autoimmune battlefield.

Chronic Pain Unveiled: Time to dive into the world of chronic pain, where everyday tasks can feel like climbing Mount Everest. We're breaking down what chronic pain is, how it messes with your mojo, and why it's time to show it who's boss.

1. **Autoimmunity Unmasked:** Ever felt like your own body was staging a rebellion? That's autoimmunity for you! Discover the inside scoop on autoimmune diseases — those sneaky troublemakers that have a party in your immune system and often leave you feeling like you've been through a real-life maze.

2. **Warrior Mode: Engaged:** We're laying it all out on the table. From the struggles of managing chronic pain to the rollercoaster ride of autoimmune flare-ups, this chapter's all about recognizing the battles we face. But guess what? We're warriors, and we're ready to tackle these challenges head-on like the legends we are. Time to suit up and face the battlefield!

    But here's the thing, understanding the enemy is the first step to victory. Knowing your adversaries inside and out empowers you to fight back smarter and stronger. So, warriors, let's dive into the facts and arm ourselves with knowledge to face these challenges head-on.

Chapter 3: The Science Behind OMAD - How It's a Total Game-Changer

Alright, it's time to geek out a bit! In this chapter, we're gonna break down the science behind OMAD like we're decoding some secret language. We'll learn how OMAD impacts our metabolism, insulin levels, and the way our bodies use energy.

OMAD ain't no fad diet, my friends. It's a lifestyle that triggers some serious body magic! So, get ready to embrace the science and understand why OMAD is about to become our BFF in this health journey!

Absolutely, I'd be happy to break down the science behind OMAD in simple terms!

Imagine your body as a car that needs fuel to run. When you eat, your body gets a supply of energy, just like putting gas in the car. But here's the cool part: when you don't eat for a while, your body starts using up the stored energy it had saved from previous meals. This stored energy comes from things like fat cells. This process is like switching from using the gas in the tank to using the gas in the trunk.

Now, OMAD takes this idea and runs with it. Instead of eating several times throughout the day, you're giving your body a longer time without food, kind of like a pit stop for the car. This longer break between meals gives your body the chance to really use up those stored energy sources. It's like your car switching to super fuel-efficient mode.

But that's not all! OMAD also gives your body a chance to regulate some important things. Like that hormone called insulin – it's like a key that lets energy into your cells. When you eat, your body releases more insulin to handle all the energy from the food. But when you do OMAD, you're not flooding your body with food all the time, so your insulin levels get a chance to chill. This can be a game-changer because it might help your body become more sensitive to insulin, which is a good thing.

And here's where the magic happens: when your body isn't constantly dealing with new energy coming in from food, it can focus on other important tasks, like cleaning up stuff that's not needed or fixing things that might be a bit wonky. It's like your car's mechanic getting to work while you're parked.

So, in a nutshell, OMAD is like giving your body a chance to use up stored energy, regulate hormones, and do some much-needed maintenance. It's a game-changer because it can help with things like having more energy, potentially managing weight, and even giving your body a chance to heal and feel better overall. It's like upgrading your car's engine to a supercharged version – you're giving your body the tools it needs to run at its best! 🚗 💧

Chapter 4: Benefits of OMAD for Chronic Pain and Autoimmune Warriors - Get Ready to Be Amazed!

Alright, squad, this chapter is where things get juicy! We're gonna talk about the fantastic benefits of OMAD that are gonna blow your mind. Say goodbye to mindless snacking and hello to improved energy levels, better mental clarity, and even potential weight loss.

OMAD is gonna help us manage inflammation, boost our immune system, and give us the upper hand in dealing with chronic pain and autoimmune flare-ups.

1. **Energy Overload:** Imagine a life where you're not constantly battling fatigue. That's the magic of OMAD, my friends! We're dishing out the deets on how OMAD can skyrocket your energy levels, making sluggishness a thing of the past.

2. **Brainpower Boost:** Say hello to mental clarity and wave goodbye to brain fog! Discover how OMAD can turn you into a cognitive superhero, helping you think sharper and brighter than ever before. Get ready to unlock your inner Einstein!

3. **Weight-Wise Wonder:** Tired of those never-ending diet rollercoasters? OMAD might just be your new bestie. Learn how it can team up with your metabolism to potentially bid farewell to those pesky pounds. It's like having a secret weight loss weapon in your pocket! Get ready to transform, warrior-style!

4. **Inflammation Buster:** Imagine taming the inflammation beast and giving your immune system a high-five. OMAD might just be the ticket! Delve into how OMAD's superhero potential could help manage inflammation and support your body's defenses, making you the ultimate immune system MVP.

5. **Warrior Wellness Unleashed:** We're not just talking about physical gains, fam. Discover how OMAD could potentially put you in the driver's seat when it comes to managing your autoimmune condition. It's like giving your body the ultimate wellness toolkit to fight back and thrive. Get ready to embrace a whole new level of warrior wellness – the OMAD way!

So, get ready to unleash the power of OMAD, 'cause we're about to step into a whole new world of health and wellness!

Chapter 5: Combining OMAD Fasting with Other Lifestyle Changes - Crafting Your Path to Wellness

Alright, it's time to level up our game! In this chapter, we're not just stopping at OMAD – we're exploring how to supercharge your journey by combining it with other lifestyle changes that'll have you feeling like an absolute boss.

Exercise and Movement for Pain Relief: Lace up those sneakers and let's get moving! Discover how incorporating regular exercise, tailored to your abilities, can help alleviate chronic pain, boost your mood, and keep your body strong and resilient.

Stress Management and Mindfulness: The mind matters, too! Dive into the world of stress management and mindfulness practices that can help you better cope with the challenges of chronic pain and autoimmunity. From meditation to deep breathing, we've got the tools to keep your mind zen.

Quality Sleep and Its Role in Healing: Get ready for some serious beauty sleep! Uncover the vital role quality sleep plays in healing and how OMAD can potentially improve your sleep patterns. We'll share tips and strategies to help you catch those Zs like a pro.

By the time you finish, you'll be equipped with a toolkit of lifestyle changes that complement your OMAD journey. These powerful additions will not only support your overall well-being but also enhance the positive impact of OMAD on your life. So, get ready to craft your unique path to wellness and unleash your inner champion!

Chapter 6: Combining OMAD Fasting with Other Lifestyle Changes

6.1 Exercise and Movement for Pain Relief

Exercise plays a crucial role in managing chronic pain and autoimmune diseases. It can help improve flexibility, strength, and overall well-being. However, it's essential to start slowly and listen to your body, especially when incorporating exercise into your routine alongside OMAD fasting. Here's a basic exercise regimen that includes walking, house chores, and cardio:

1. Daily Walking: Walking is a low-impact exercise that can be easily incorporated into your daily routine. It helps improve circulation, maintain joint mobility, and boost your mood. Start with a 10-15 minute walk every day and gradually increase the duration as you feel comfortable.

- Tips:
- Find a scenic route or a local park to make walking more enjoyable.
- Consider walking with a friend or family member for motivation and support.

2. Active House Chores: Believe it or not, household chores can be an excellent way to stay active and burn calories. Engage in tasks that involve movement, such as vacuuming, mopping, gardening, or washing windows.

- Tips:
- Break down chores into smaller tasks and take short breaks between them.
- Focus on maintaining good posture to avoid straining your back or joints.

3. Cardio Exercises: Cardiovascular exercises help improve heart health and stamina. Depending on your fitness level, you can choose from various options such as cycling, swimming, dancing, or using a stationary bike.

- Tips:
- Start with 10-15 minutes of cardio and gradually increase the duration.
- Consider low-impact options if you have joint issues or chronic pain.

Remember, the key is to find activities that you enjoy and that suit your body's capabilities. Always consult with your healthcare provider before starting any new exercise regimen, especially if you have specific health concerns or conditions.

It's important to note that exercising while fasting may require some adjustments. If you prefer to exercise during your fasting period, opt for low-intensity activities like walking or light stretching. On the other hand, if you feel more energetic after your meal, schedule your exercise routine accordingly.

Stay hydrated during exercise, and don't push yourself too hard, especially if you're just starting. Gradually increase the intensity and duration of your workouts as your body becomes accustomed to the exercise regimen.

By combining the benefits of OMAD fasting with regular exercise, you can create a holistic approach to managing chronic pain and autoimmune diseases. Exercise not only aids in pain relief but also contributes to your overall physical and mental well-being. Always listen to your body, respect your limitations, and celebrate your progress along the way.

6.2 Stress Management and Mindfulness

Chronic pain and autoimmune disorders can be exacerbated by stress and worry. Stress management and mindfulness practice can have a big impact on your overall well-being. Here's how to include stress-reduction techniques into your daily routine.:

1. Mindfulness Meditation:

- Practice mindfulness meditation to stay present and reduce stress levels.
- Use guided meditation apps or attend meditation classes for support.

2. Breathing Exercises:

- Practice deep breathing exercises to calm the nervous system and reduce stress.
- Try techniques like diaphragmatic breathing and alternate nostril breathing.

3. Relaxation Techniques:

- Engage in activities that promote relaxation, such as reading, listening to music, or spending time in nature.
- Consider activities that bring you joy and peace of mind.

4. Time Management:

- Create a balanced daily schedule that includes time for rest, work, exercise, and relaxation.
- Avoid overcommitting and learn to say no when needed.

6.3 Quality Sleep and Its Role in Healing

Getting enough quality sleep is critical for your overall health and well-being, particularly if you suffer from chronic pain or autoimmune illnesses. A regular sleep schedule can aid with pain management as well as prevent late-night snacking, which can interrupt your fasting regimen. Here's a sleep regimen that encourages peaceful sleep while decreasing late-night desires:

1. Set a Consistent Bedtime: Try to go to bed and wake up at the same time every day, even on weekends. Consistency helps regulate your internal clock, making it easier to fall asleep and wake up naturally.

2. Create a Relaxing Bedtime Routine: Establish a calming routine before bedtime to signal your body that it's time to wind down. This could include activities such as reading a book, taking a warm bath, practicing gentle stretching or meditation, or listening to soothing music.

3. Limit Screen Time Before Bed: The blue light emitted by screens can interfere with your sleep cycle. Try to avoid screens (phones, tablets, computers, and TVs) at least an hour before bedtime.

4. Make Your Bedroom Sleep-Friendly: Create a sleep-conducive environment in your bedroom. Keep the room cool, dark, and quiet. Invest in comfortable bedding and a supportive mattress to improve your sleep quality.

5. Avoid Heavy Meals and Stimulants Before Bed: Refrain from consuming heavy meals or stimulants like caffeine and nicotine close to bedtime. These can disrupt your ability to fall asleep and stay asleep.

6. Manage Stress and Anxiety: Practicing relaxation techniques or mindfulness exercises during the day can help reduce stress and anxiety, promoting better sleep at night.

7. Stay Active During the Day: Regular physical activity can improve sleep quality. However, avoid intense exercise close to bedtime, as it may make falling asleep more challenging.

8.   Snack Mindfully or Opt for Herbal Tea: If you feel the urge to snack late at night, choose light and healthy options or opt for a cup of herbal tea. Avoid sugary or high-calorie snacks that can interfere with your fasting goals.

9.   Avoid Long Naps: While short power naps can be refreshing, long naps during the day might disrupt your nighttime sleep. If you need to nap, limit it to 20-30 minutes.

10.   Keep a Sleep Journal: Keep track of your sleep patterns, including bedtime, wake-up time, and any factors that may affect your sleep. This can help identify patterns and adjustments needed for better sleep quality.

By following a consistent sleep schedule and creating a relaxing bedtime routine, you can improve your sleep quality and reduce the likelihood of late-night snacking. Quality sleep is a vital component of the healing process and complements the benefits of OMAD fasting in managing chronic pain and autoimmune diseases. Aim for 7-9 hours of sleep per night, and remember that getting adequate rest is an essential part of your holistic approach to wellness.

Chapter 7: Troubleshooting and Overcoming Challenges

7.1 Dealing with Plateaus

It's common to experience plateaus while on the OMAD fasting journey. Plateaus occur when your body adapts to the new eating pattern, and weight loss or health improvements slow down. Here's how to overcome plateaus and continue progressing:

1.   Mix Up Your Meals:

•   Experiment with different foods and meal combinations to keep your metabolism active.

•   Include a variety of nutrients in your OMAD meals, such as lean proteins, healthy fats, and fiber-rich vegetables.

2.   Introduce Intermittent Fasting Variations:

•   Consider incorporating intermittent fasting variations like 16/8 (16 hours fasting, 8 hours eating window) or 5:2 (eating normally for 5 days, fasting or eating very few calories for 2 non-consecutive days).

3.   Increase Physical Activity:

• Boost your activity level with new exercises or increase the intensity of your current workout routine.

• Physical activity can help break through plateaus by increasing calorie expenditure.

4. Reassess Your Caloric Intake:

• Ensure you're not consuming too many calories during your OMAD meal.

• Use portion control and mindful eating to avoid overeating.

5. Stay Patient and Persistent:

• Plateaus are a normal part of any health journey. Stay committed and patient, and remember that progress may not always be linear.

7.2 Common Fasting Side Effects and How to Address Them

Fasting may initially cause some side effects as your body adjusts to the new eating pattern. Here are common side effects and how to address them:

1. Hunger Pangs:

• Stay well-hydrated and consume calorie-free beverages like water, herbal tea, or black coffee to help reduce hunger.

2. Fatigue:

• Ensure you're getting enough sleep and rest.

• Consume nutrient-dense foods during your OMAD meal to maintain energy levels.

3. Headaches:

• Headaches are often a sign of dehydration. Drink plenty of water throughout the day to stay hydrated.

4. Dizziness or Lightheadedness:

• If you experience

Chapter 8: Mindful Eating on OMAD - Savoring Every Bite

Get ready to transform your relationship with food as we dive into the art of mindful eating within the OMAD framework. In this chapter, we're shifting gears from just what you eat to how you eat, unlocking a whole new level of awareness and satisfaction.

The Power of Mindful Eating: Brace yourself for a game-changer! Learn how mindful eating can transform your OMAD experience by fostering a deeper connection with your body and its hunger cues. We'll guide you through the process of being present in the moment, making each meal a truly enriching experience.

Avoiding Emotional Eating Traps: We've all been there – stress, boredom, or emotions triggering those unwelcome food cravings. Discover effective strategies to navigate emotional eating pitfalls, ensuring that your OMAD journey remains focused on nourishment rather than coping with emotions.

Mindful Eating Tips for OMAD Success: Time to get practical! We're dishing out actionable tips and techniques to incorporate mindful eating into your OMAD routine. From setting the stage for mealtime to engaging your senses, you'll have a toolkit to make each OMAD meal a mindful feast.

By the time you finish this chapter, you'll have the tools to transform your OMAD meals into moments of mindfulness and joy. Get ready to savor every bite, embrace a new level of food appreciation, and elevate your OMAD experience to a whole new level of nourishment and self-awareness. Let's dive in and make mindful eating a cornerstone of your OMAD success!

Absolutely, hydration is essential, and incorporating herbal teas and fruit-infused water can be a fantastic addition to your daily routine. Not only do they help prevent unnecessary snacking, but they also offer a variety of health benefits, including detoxification and an added dose of vitamins and minerals. Let's explore these refreshing options:

1. Herbal Teas for Detoxification:

Herbal teas are a wonderful way to support your body's natural detoxification process and provide soothing hydration. Here are some popular herbal teas known for their detoxifying properties:

- Green Tea: Packed with antioxidants, green tea helps boost metabolism and aids in flushing out toxins from the body.

- Dandelion Root Tea: Known for its liver-cleansing properties, dandelion root tea can support your body's detoxification pathways.

- Peppermint Tea: Not only does peppermint tea have a calming effect on the digestive system, but it can also aid in eliminating waste and toxins from the body.

- Ginger Tea: Ginger is well-known for its anti-inflammatory properties and can help improve digestion and detoxification.

- Nettle Tea: Nettle tea acts as a diuretic, supporting kidney function and promoting detoxification through urine flow.

2. Fruit-Infused Water for Added Vitamins and Minerals:

Fruit-infused water is a delightful and flavorful way to stay hydrated while also benefiting from the vitamins and minerals present in the fruits. Here's how to prepare it:

- Choose your favorite fruits and herbs (e.g., berries, citrus slices, cucumber, mint) and wash them thoroughly.

- Slice the fruits or herbs and add them to a pitcher or large water bottle.

- Fill the container with water and refrigerate for at least a few hours to allow the flavors to infuse.

- Sip on this refreshing fruit-infused water throughout the day to stay hydrated and get a boost of nutrients.

By incorporating herbal teas and fruit-infused water into your daily routine, you not only stay hydrated but also enjoy the added benefits of detoxification and a nutrient boost. These flavorful alternatives can help curb cravings and prevent snacking, supporting your OMAD fasting journey and overall health. Cheers to a tasty and nourishing way to stay on track!

Storytime

Alright, let me share a real-life story that's straight outta my own experience with OMAD – no sugar-coating, just the raw truth.

So, picture this: a few years back, I decided to jump on the OMAD bandwagon to deal with my chronic pain and autoimmune issues. I was pumped and ready to embrace this trendy fasting lifestyle. My first few days were exciting; I felt like a boss, conquering hunger like a warrior.

But, here comes the plot twist — I hit a major bump in the road. My body rebelled, and I started feeling hangry all the time. My energy levels dipped, and I had headaches that could knock a bear off its feet. I won't lie; it was rough as hell, and I felt like giving up. I thought, "OMAD ain't for me; I can't handle this!"

But, I ain't no quitter. I dusted myself off, did some research, and realized I made some rookie mistakes. I wasn't drinking enough water and ended up dehydrated AF. I was also eating junk during my one meal, thinking it was all about the calories.

So, I hit the reset button and started over — this time, with a fresh mindset and a badass plan. I upped my water game, and guess what? Those hangry vibes disappeared like magic. I replaced the junk with wholesome, nutrient-rich foods during my OMAD feast and boom! The headaches went poof!

Now, I ain't gonna lie, it wasn't all rainbows and unicorns. I still faced challenges, and there were days when I slipped back into old habits. But, here's the thing — I never gave up! I'd brush off the setbacks and get back on the OMAD train. I mean, ain't nobody's journey perfect, right?

Slowly but surely, things started falling into place. My energy skyrocketed, and I felt more in control of my body than ever. My chronic pain began to ease up, and my autoimmune flare-ups became less frequent. It was like a damn miracle!

Sure, it took time, commitment, and a whole lotta patience, but I learned one valuable lesson — persistence pays off! So, here I am, embracing the OMAD lifestyle like a boss, and I'm never looking back.

Life's all about the ups and downs, but I'm determined to stay on this path and keep rocking OMAD. No matter how many times I stumble, I'll always rise up, because giving up ain't my style, fam.

So, if you're starting your own OMAD journey or facing struggles, remember this tale of mine. It's okay to have hiccups; just don't let 'em define you. Keep hustling, keep learning, and keep slaying those goals — you got this! 💪✨

Yo, let me drop some real talk here! So, about two years ago, I decided to take control of my life and jump on the OMAD train. But here's the kicker – I was pushing almost 300 pounds on the scale! Yeah, you heard that right – a whole lotta extra me.

I was fed up with feeling sluggish, dealing with chronic pain, and battling those annoying autoimmune flare-ups. So, I thought, "Hey, maybe OMAD's the answer to all my prayers!" I dove in headfirst, excited to see some real results.

And you know what? It worked! The first time around, I lost around 30 to 40 pounds like a boss! I was on cloud nine, feeling like I could take on the world. But, oh boy, life had other plans for me.

I hit a plateau, and BAM! The weight started creeping back up like it had its own agenda. It was frustrating as hell, and I felt like a failure. But I ain't one to back down easily. I got back on track and lost those same 30 to 40 pounds all over again.

But guess what? History repeated itself, and I faced another setback. You might be thinking, "Damn, did you ever find your groove?" Oh, you bet I did, my friend!

See, I learned from each hiccup, each stumble, and each time I hit a roadblock. I realized that my approach needed tweaking. It wasn't just about shedding pounds; it was about finding my perfect OMAD schedule.

So, I took a deep breath, wiped away those tears of frustration, and got back into the game. I experimented with different eating windows, meal choices, and exercise routines. And finally, after a whole lot of trial and error, it happened – I found my sweet spot!

I hit that magical stride where OMAD became my lifestyle, not just a diet. It was like a switch flipped, and everything fell into place. The weight started coming off steadily, my chronic pain eased up, and my autoimmune flare-ups showed up less and less.

It's been a journey of ups and downs, and I've had to lose those same 30 to 40 pounds over and over again. But you know what? I ain't mad about it. It taught me resilience, patience, and the power of never giving up on myself.

So, here I am today, continuing to make strides on my OMAD journey. I might've started at almost 300 pounds, but I'm moving forward with my head held high, knowing I've got the strength to conquer whatever comes my way.

If you're starting your own OMAD path or struggling with setbacks, remember my story. It ain't about the number on the scale or how many times you stumble. It's about the grit in your soul and the determination to keep pushing forward, no matter what.

You got this, fam – the power to rise above, find your groove, and embrace your own OMAD magic! 🌟 💪

Extra tips

Embracing One Meal a Day (OMAD) fasting doesn't mean you have to miss out on enjoying meals with family and friends. Here are some creative ways to eat with your loved ones while staying true to your OMAD fasting routine:

1. Host a Themed Potluck: Organize a potluck with a specific theme, such as international cuisines, comfort foods, or healthy dishes. Each person can contribute a dish that aligns with your dietary preferences and OMAD fasting goals.

2. Cook Together: Invite your family and friends to cook together in the kitchen. While they prepare their meals, you can participate by preparing your OMAD meal. It becomes an enjoyable and communal cooking experience.

3. OMAD Picnic: Plan an outdoor picnic where everyone brings their own meal. You can still enjoy each other's company while savoring your OMAD meal in a beautiful natural setting.

4. Family Recipe Challenge: Challenge your loved ones to create OMAD-friendly versions of their favorite family recipes. You can all taste and compare the different dishes and share in the joy of experimenting with new flavors.

5. Share Your OMAD Journey: Take the opportunity to educate your family and friends about OMAD fasting and its benefits. When they understand your choice, they may become more supportive and interested in joining you for meals.

6.   Appreciate the Social Aspect: Focus on the social interactions and connections during mealtime rather than solely on the food. Engage in meaningful conversations and enjoy the company of your loved ones.

7.   Opt for Flexible OMAD Days: If you have a special occasion or a family gathering where you'd like to eat together, consider having flexible OMAD days. Adjust your fasting window to accommodate the event without compromising your overall progress.

8.   Arrange Brunch or Lunch Gatherings: If OMAD dinner conflicts with most social gatherings, consider shifting your fasting window to enjoy a shared brunch or lunch with family and friends.

9.   Be Open About Your Needs: Communicate your OMAD schedule and goals to your loved ones. By being open about your preferences, they can better support you in finding appropriate mealtime solutions.

Remember that the essence of sharing meals with family and friends lies in the bond and joy of being together. OMAD fasting is a flexible approach, and with some creativity and communication, you can enjoy the company of your loved ones while staying committed to your health and wellness journey.

Absolutely! When dealing with chronic pain, especially on days when getting out of bed might feel challenging, exercises that can be performed from the bed can be incredibly helpful in maintaining mobility and reducing discomfort. These bed exercises are gentle on the body and can be tailored to your specific pain levels and physical abilities. Here are some bed exercises that can aid in maintaining mobility and improving flexibility:

1.   Gentle Leg Lifts:
- Lie flat on your back with your legs extended.
- Slowly lift one leg off the bed, keeping it straight, and hold for a few seconds.
- Lower the leg back down and repeat with the other leg.
- Aim for 10-15 repetitions on each leg.

2.   Ankle Circles:

- Lie on your back with your legs extended.
- Lift one leg slightly off the bed and rotate your ankle in circular motions.
- Perform 10 circles in one direction and then switch to the other direction.
- Repeat with the other leg.

3. Knee-to-Chest Stretch:
- Lie on your back with your legs extended.
- Bring one knee towards your chest, holding it with both hands.
- Hold the stretch for 15-30 seconds, feeling the gentle stretch in your lower back and hip.
- Release and repeat with the other leg.

4. Abdominal Contractions:
- Lie on your back with your knees bent and feet flat on the bed.
- Tighten your abdominal muscles as if pulling your belly button towards your spine.
- Hold the contraction for 5-10 seconds and release.
- Repeat for 10-15 repetitions.

5. Seated Arm Raises:
- Sit up in bed with your back supported by pillows.
- Hold a lightweight water bottle in each hand.
- Raise your arms up to shoulder height and then lower them back down.
- Aim for 10-15 repetitions.

Remember to breathe deeply and maintain a comfortable pace throughout these exercises. Listen to your body and adjust the range of motion or intensity as needed to avoid any exacerbation of pain. If any exercise causes discomfort, stop immediately and consult with your healthcare provider.

Bed exercises are a great option for maintaining mobility on days when you may be experiencing more pain or fatigue. Incorporating these gentle movements into your daily routine can contribute to improved flexibility, better circulation, and overall well-being while dealing with chronic pain. Always prioritize your comfort and safety, and know that even small movements can make a significant difference in your mobility and pain management.

Chapter 9: The Social Aspect of OMAD - Navigating Family and Social Gatherings

You hit the nail on the head! Online friendships and finding communities of like-minded individuals who practice OMAD can be a game-changer when it comes to staying motivated, discovering new recipes, and finding the encouragement you need on your journey. While our family and friends may have the best intentions, they might not fully understand or support our lifestyle choices in the long run. That's where online OMAD communities come to the rescue! Let's dive into why these virtual friendships are so awesome:

1.	Recipe Exchange and Inspiration:

•	Online OMAD groups are a treasure trove of delicious and creative recipes. Members love sharing their favorite OMAD meals, snacks, and treats that cater to various dietary preferences and restrictions.

•	Discovering new recipes keeps your meals exciting and diverse, making it easier to stick to your OMAD routine with enthusiasm.

2.	Encouragement and Accountability:

•	OMAD can be both physically and mentally challenging, especially during tough moments. Being part of a supportive online community means having a group of individuals who understand your struggles and celebrate your successes.

•	Members offer encouragement, share their own experiences, and provide tips to help you stay on track with your goals.

3.	Understanding and Empathy:

- Sometimes, it's tough for family and friends to grasp the intricacies of OMAD and its impact on our lives. Online OMAD communities are filled with people who face similar challenges and victories.

- The understanding and empathy you receive in these groups create a safe space where you can share your journey without judgment.

4. Motivation and Inspiration:

- Seeing the progress and achievements of others in the community can be incredibly motivating. Witnessing their transformations and reading success stories can inspire you to keep pushing forward and embrace the OMAD lifestyle wholeheartedly.

5. Access to Resources and Information:

- Online OMAD communities are a treasure trove of information and resources. From expert advice to research-backed articles, you'll find valuable insights to enhance your understanding of OMAD and its potential benefits.

6. Making Friends from Around the Globe:

- The beauty of online friendships is that they know no geographical boundaries. Connecting with people from different cultures and backgrounds who share a common interest can broaden your horizons and enrich your experience.

Chapter 10: Celebrating Progress and Staying Motivated - Unleash Your Inner Warrior

Alright, fellow warriors, it's time to throw some confetti in the air and celebrate your wins like there's no tomorrow! In this final chapter, we're diving deep into the art of celebrating progress, finding motivation in unexpected places, and keeping that fire burning bright on your OMAD journey.

Recognizing Non-Scale Victories: It's not just about the numbers, fam! Learn to recognize and celebrate those victories that don't involve the scale. From improved energy levels to hitting a new personal best in your workouts, we're all about celebrating those non-scale triumphs like the champs we are.

The Power of Progress Photos: Say cheese, because we're about to unlock the magic of progress photos! We'll guide you through the process of capturing your journey visually, giving you a powerful tool to track your transformation and stay motivated like a true superstar.

Creating a Supportive OMAD Community: It's all about the squad! Discover the incredible impact of building a supportive OMAD community around you. Whether it's online buddies, workout partners, or friends who share your OMAD journey, having a crew that cheers you on can make all the difference.

So, here's the deal, warriors — by the time you finish this chapter, you'll be armed with a toolkit of celebration, motivation, and community-building strategies that'll have you embracing your OMAD journey with fierce determination. Get ready to unleash your inner warrior, celebrate every step of the way, and keep the OMAD flame burning as bright as ever. You've got this, and the world better be ready for the unstoppable force that you've become!

Remember, everyone's journey is unique, and it's okay to seek support beyond your immediate circle. Online friendships in OMAD communities offer a sense of belonging and camaraderie that can be incredibly empowering on your path to better health and well-being. So, dive in, engage, and make the most of this incredible opportunity to connect with OMAD enthusiasts who will cheer you on every step of the way! 💝 💪

Shopping List

Name:
- [ ]
- [ ]
- [ ]
- [ ]
- [ ]
- [ ]
- [ ]
- [ ]
- [ ]
- [ ]
- [ ]
- [ ]
- [ ]
- [ ]
- [ ]

Name:
- [ ]
- [ ]
- [ ]
- [ ]
- [ ]
- [ ]
- [ ]
- [ ]
- [ ]
- [ ]
- [ ]
- [ ]
- [ ]
- [ ]
- [ ]

Name:
- [ ]
- [ ]
- [ ]
- [ ]
- [ ]
- [ ]
- [ ]
- [ ]
- [ ]
- [ ]
- [ ]
- [ ]
- [ ]
- [ ]
- [ ]

Name:
- [ ]
- [ ]
- [ ]
- [ ]
- [ ]
- [ ]
- [ ]
- [ ]
- [ ]
- [ ]
- [ ]
- [ ]
- [ ]
- [ ]
- [ ]

Shopping List

Name:

Name:

Name:

Name:

Shopping List

Name:

Name:

Name:

Name:

Shopping List

Name:

Name:

Name:

Name:

Shopping List

Name:

Name:

Name:

Name:

Shopping List

Name:
☐
☐
☐
☐
☐
☐
☐
☐
☐
☐
☐
☐
☐
☐
☐

Name:
☐
☐
☐
☐
☐
☐
☐
☐
☐
☐
☐
☐
☐
☐
☐

Name:
☐
☐
☐
☐
☐
☐
☐
☐
☐
☐
☐
☐
☐
☐
☐

Name:
☐
☐
☐
☐
☐
☐
☐
☐
☐
☐
☐
☐
☐
☐
☐

Shopping List

Name:
- [ ]
- [ ]
- [ ]
- [ ]
- [ ]
- [ ]
- [ ]
- [ ]
- [ ]
- [ ]
- [ ]
- [ ]
- [ ]
- [ ]
- [ ]

Name:
- [ ]
- [ ]
- [ ]
- [ ]
- [ ]
- [ ]
- [ ]
- [ ]
- [ ]
- [ ]
- [ ]
- [ ]
- [ ]
- [ ]
- [ ]

Name:
- [ ]
- [ ]
- [ ]
- [ ]
- [ ]
- [ ]
- [ ]
- [ ]
- [ ]
- [ ]
- [ ]
- [ ]
- [ ]
- [ ]
- [ ]

Name:
- [ ]
- [ ]
- [ ]
- [ ]
- [ ]
- [ ]
- [ ]
- [ ]
- [ ]
- [ ]
- [ ]
- [ ]
- [ ]
- [ ]
- [ ]

Shopping List

Name:
- [ ]
- [ ]
- [ ]
- [ ]
- [ ]
- [ ]
- [ ]
- [ ]
- [ ]
- [ ]
- [ ]
- [ ]
- [ ]
- [ ]
- [ ]

Name:
- [ ]
- [ ]
- [ ]
- [ ]
- [ ]
- [ ]
- [ ]
- [ ]
- [ ]
- [ ]
- [ ]
- [ ]
- [ ]
- [ ]
- [ ]

Name:
- [ ]
- [ ]
- [ ]
- [ ]
- [ ]
- [ ]
- [ ]
- [ ]
- [ ]
- [ ]
- [ ]
- [ ]
- [ ]
- [ ]
- [ ]

Name:
- [ ]
- [ ]
- [ ]
- [ ]
- [ ]
- [ ]
- [ ]
- [ ]
- [ ]
- [ ]
- [ ]
- [ ]
- [ ]
- [ ]
- [ ]

Shopping List

Name:

Name:

Name:

Name:

Shopping List

Name:

Name:

Name:

Name:

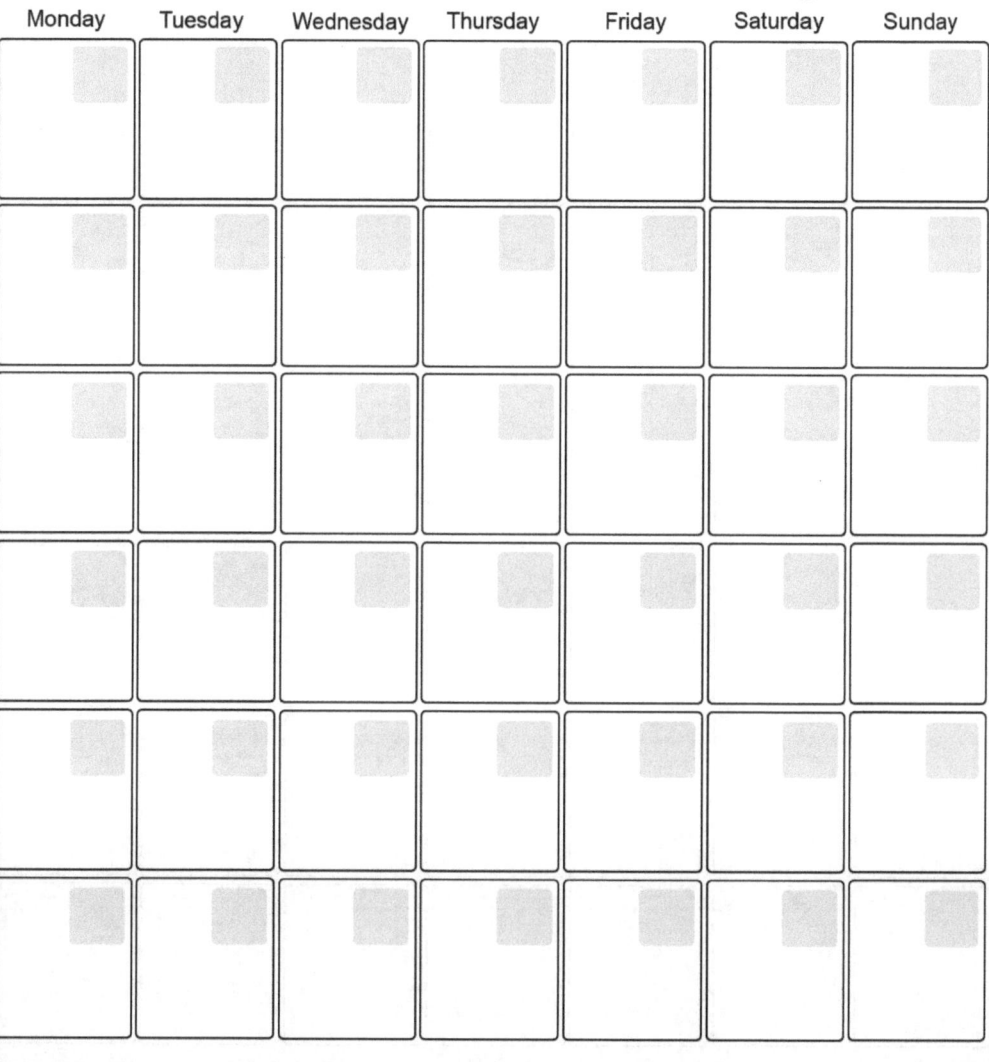

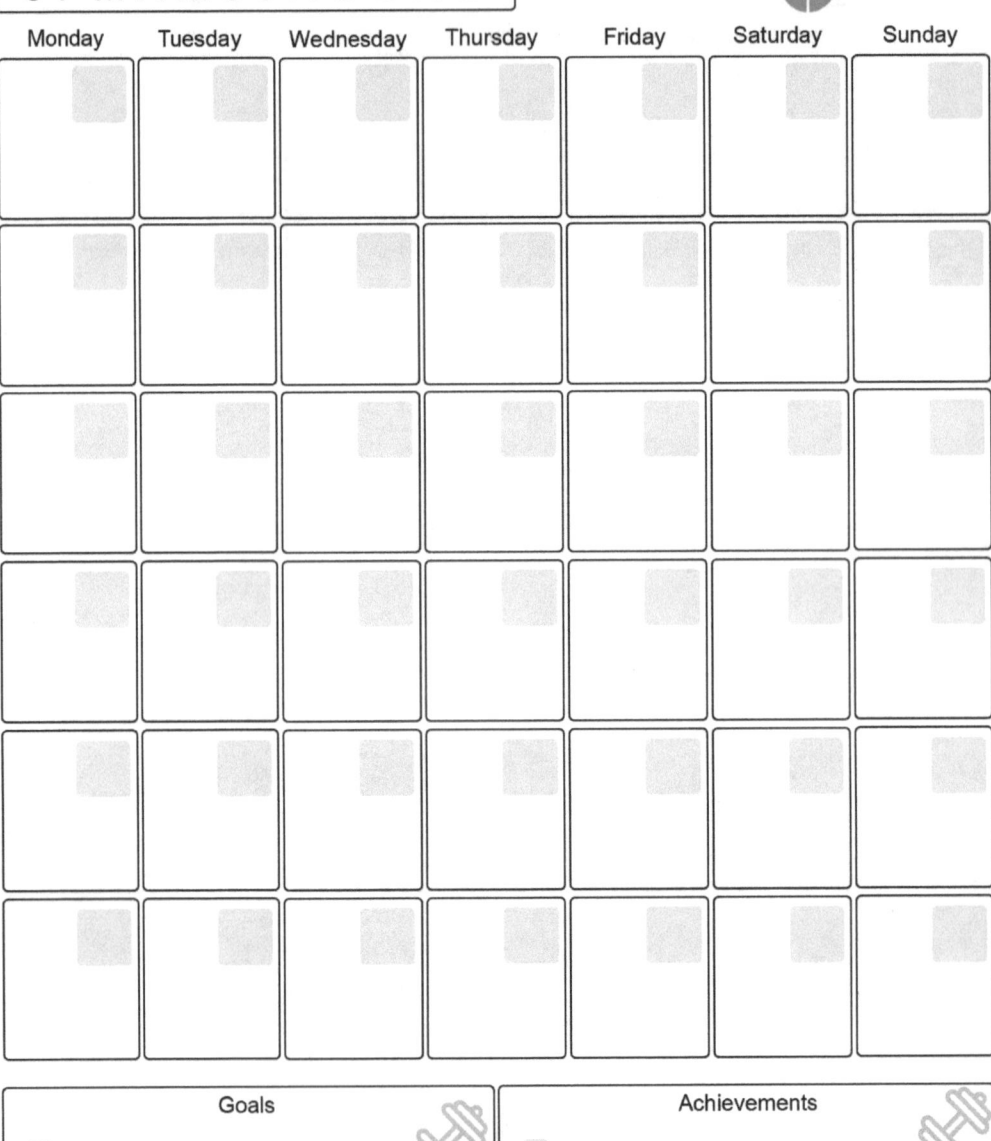

Fitness Calendar

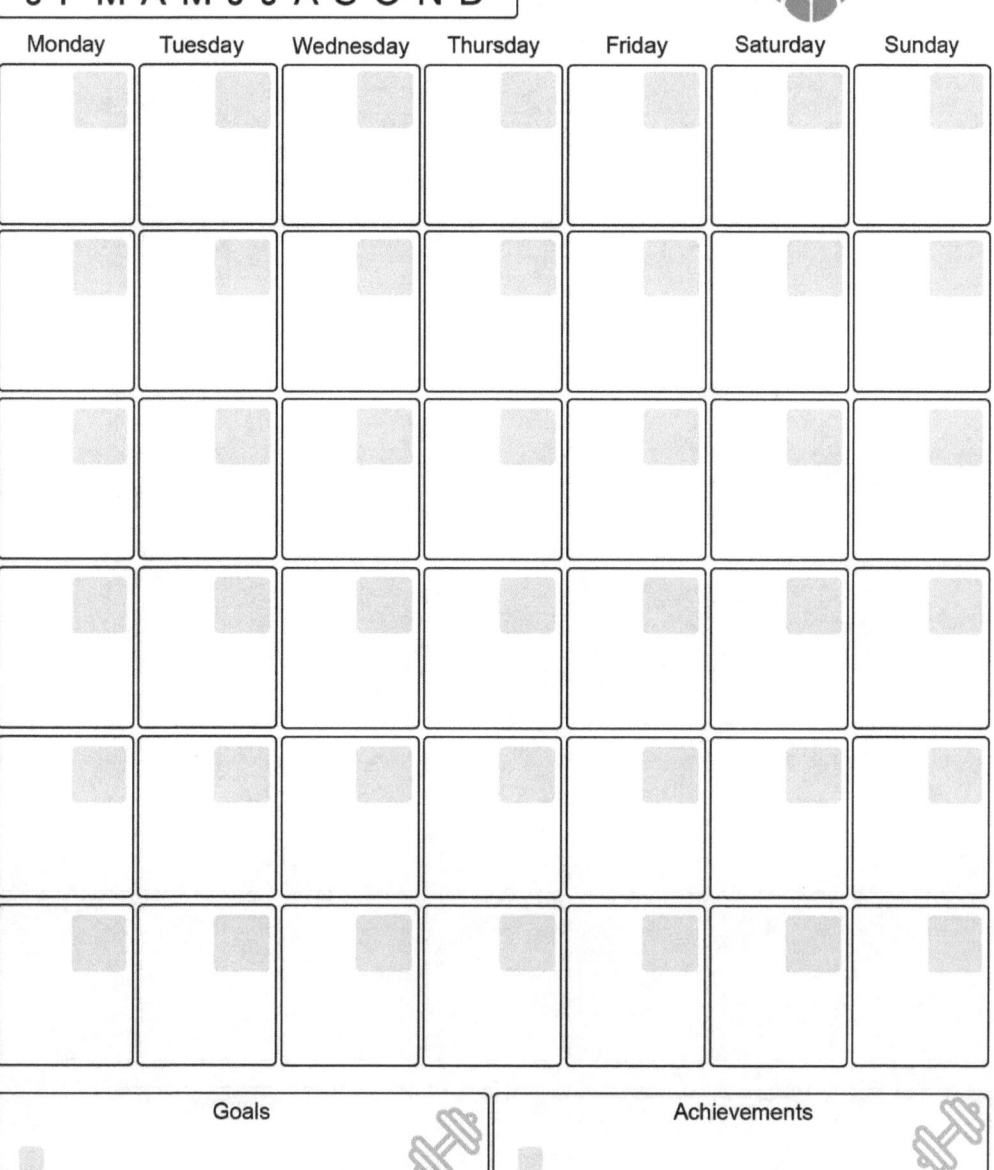

Year:

J F M A M J J A S O N D

Monday	Tuesday	Wednesday	Thursday	Friday	Saturday	Sunday

Goals

Achievements

Fitness Calendar

Year:

J F M A M J J A S O N D

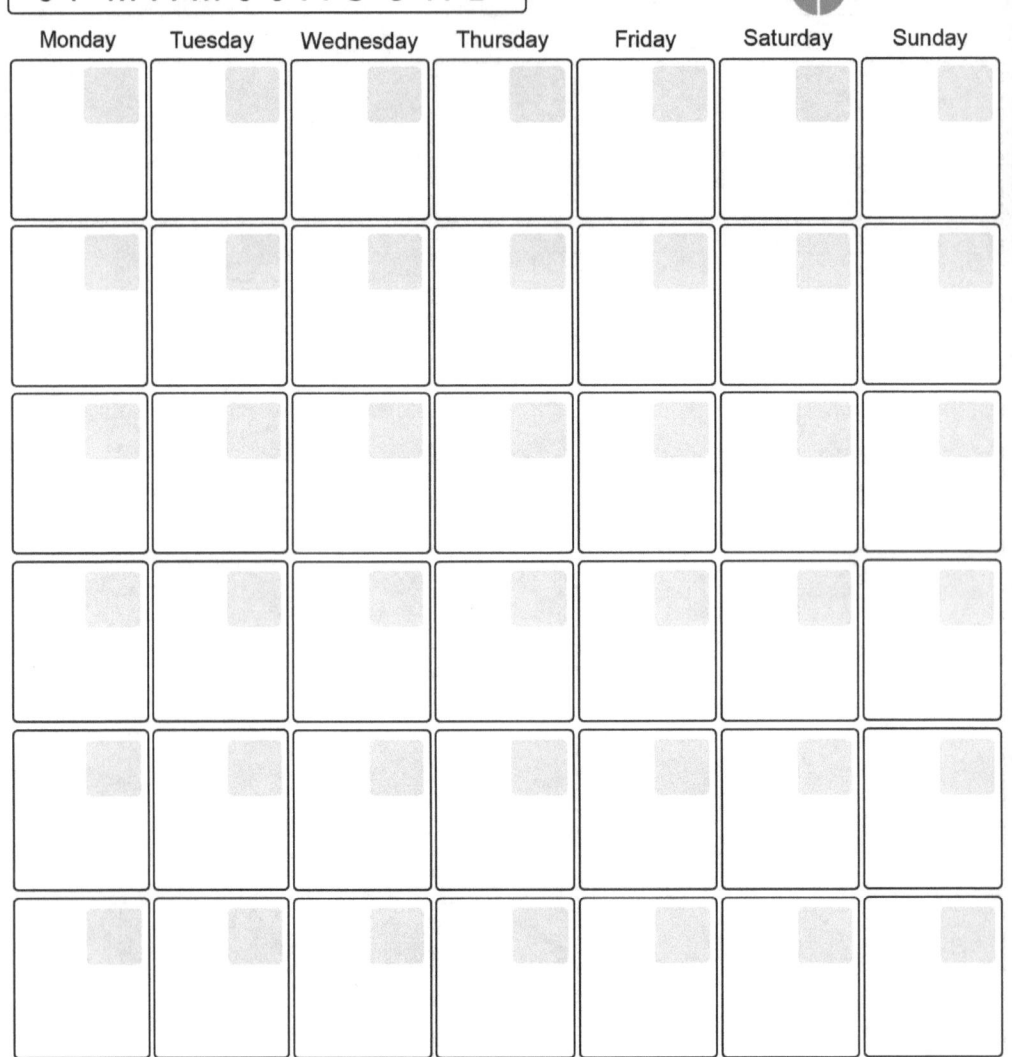

Monday	Tuesday	Wednesday	Thursday	Friday	Saturday	Sunday

Goals	Achievements

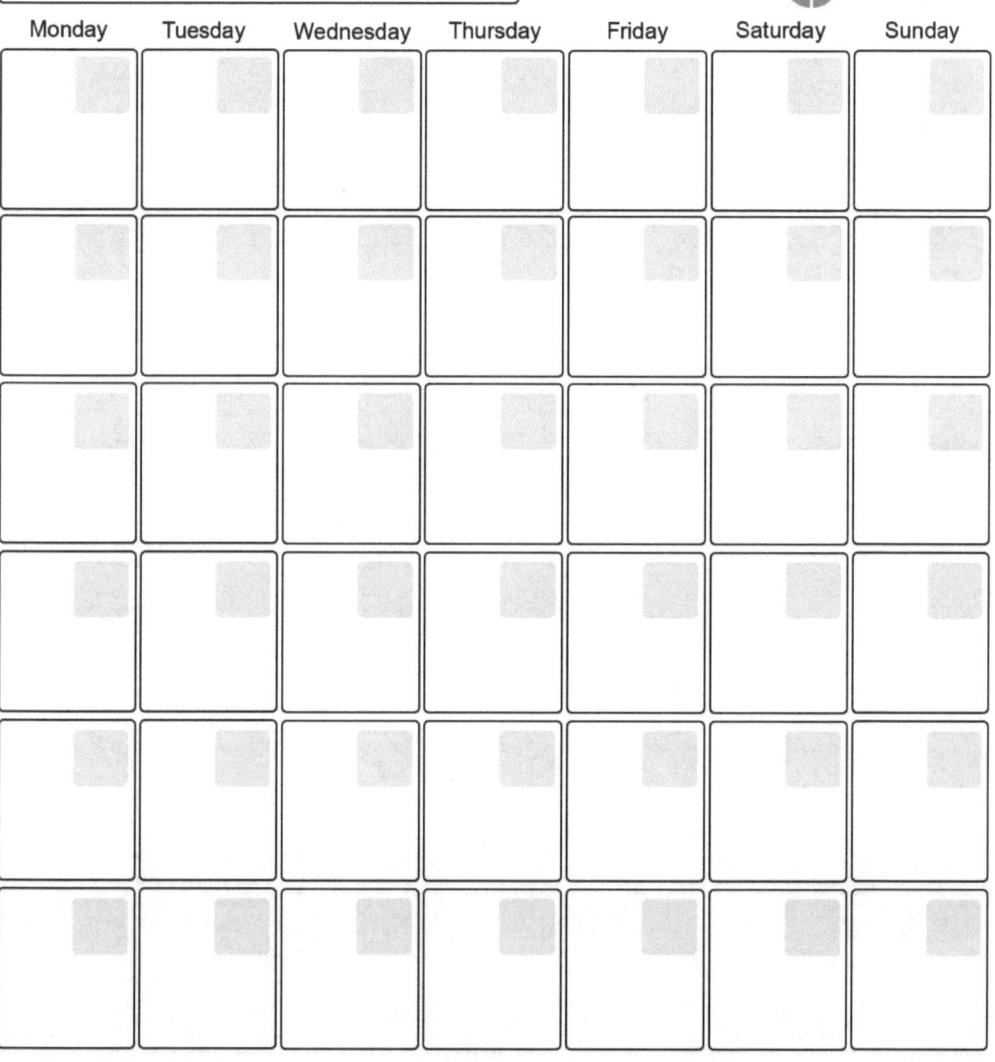

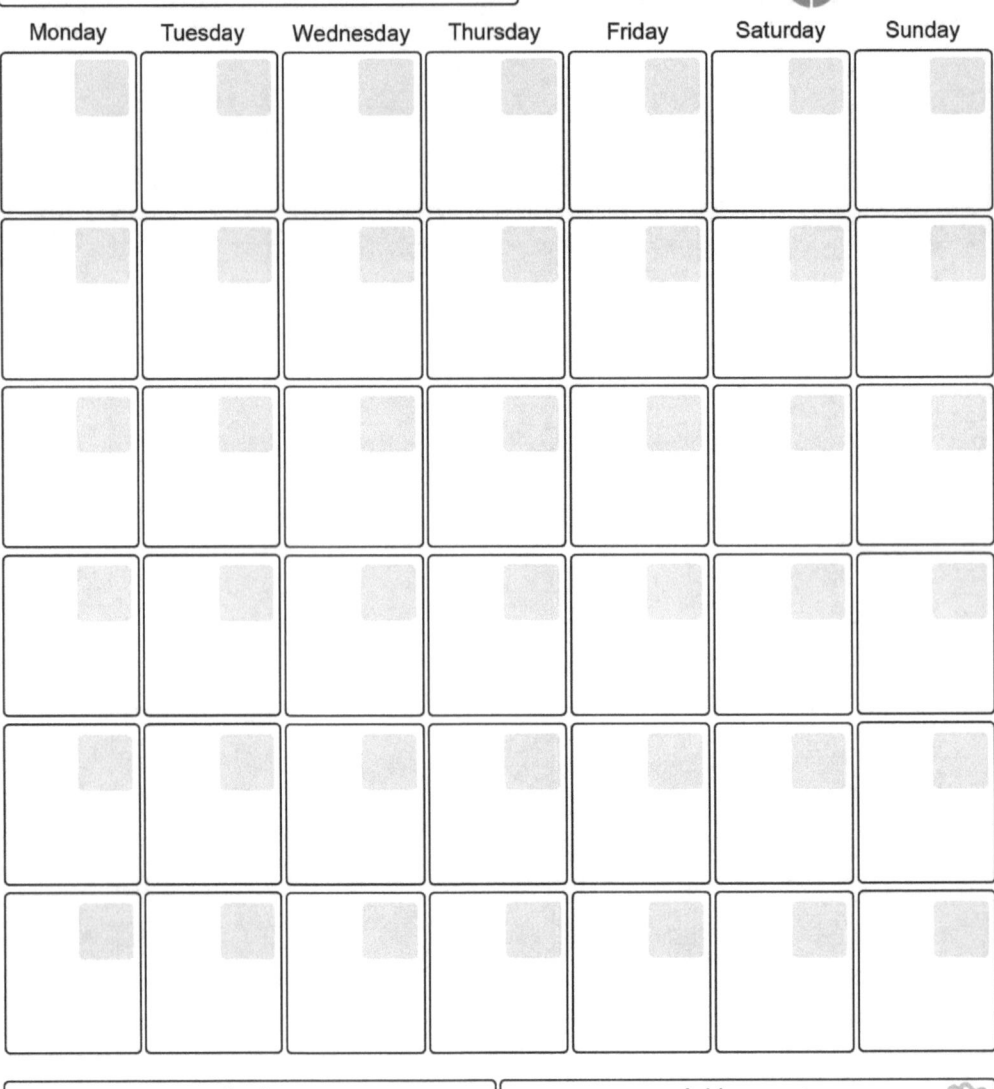

Fitness Calendar

Year:

J F M A M J J A S O N D

Monday	Tuesday	Wednesday	Thursday	Friday	Saturday	Sunday

Goals

Achievements

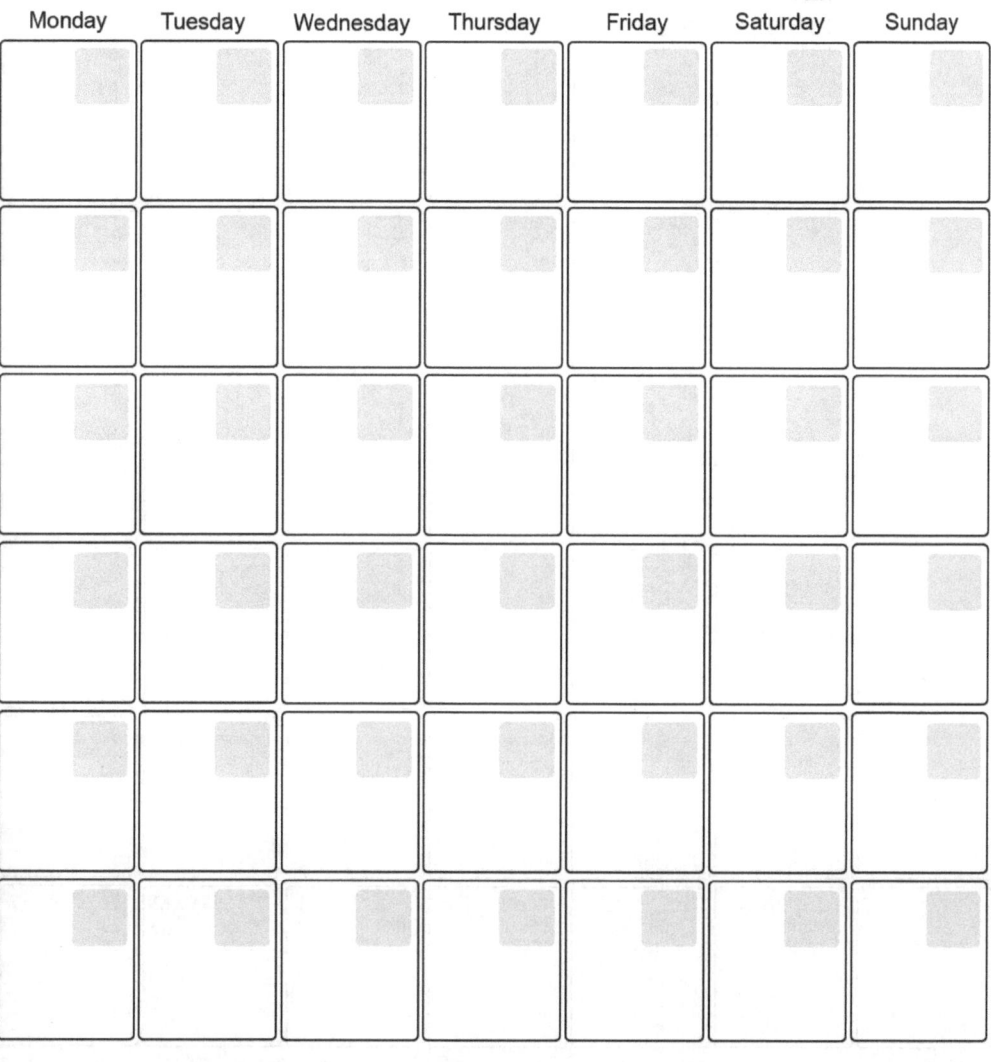

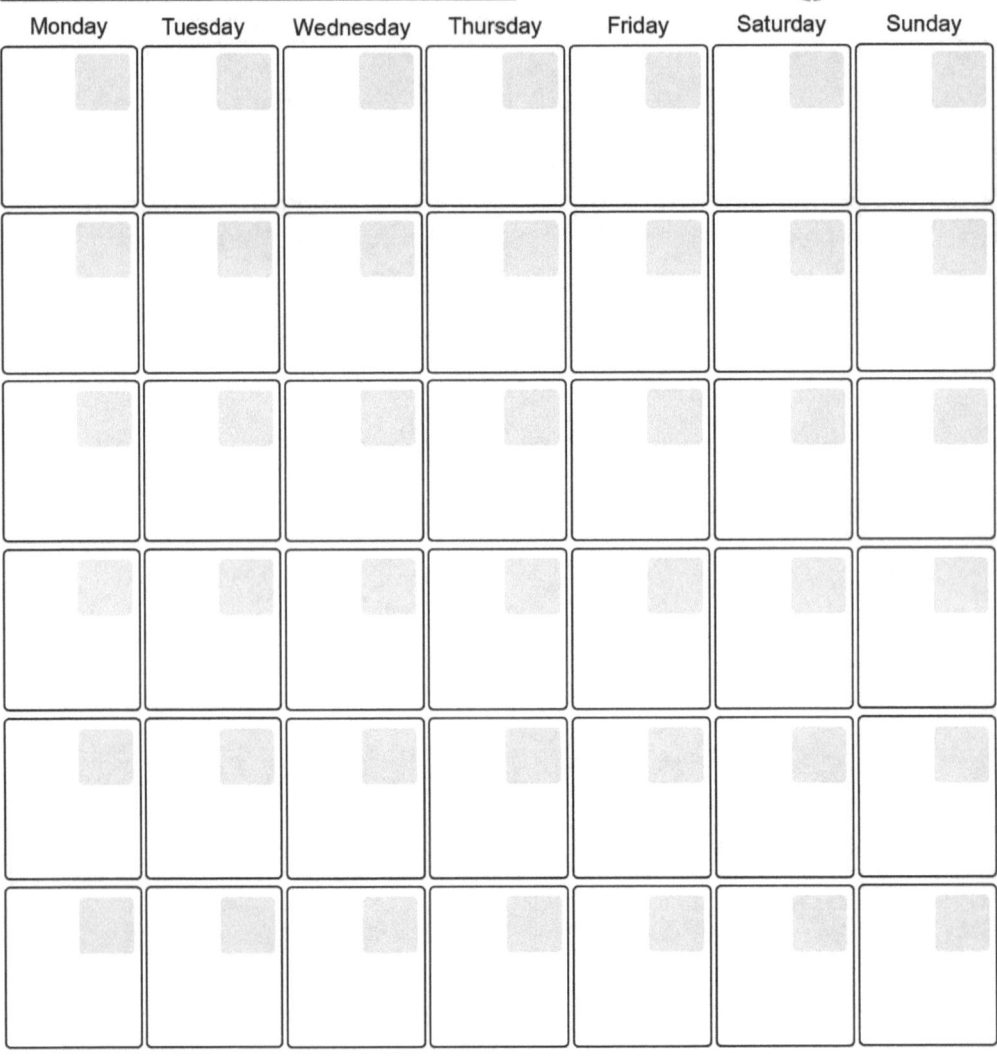

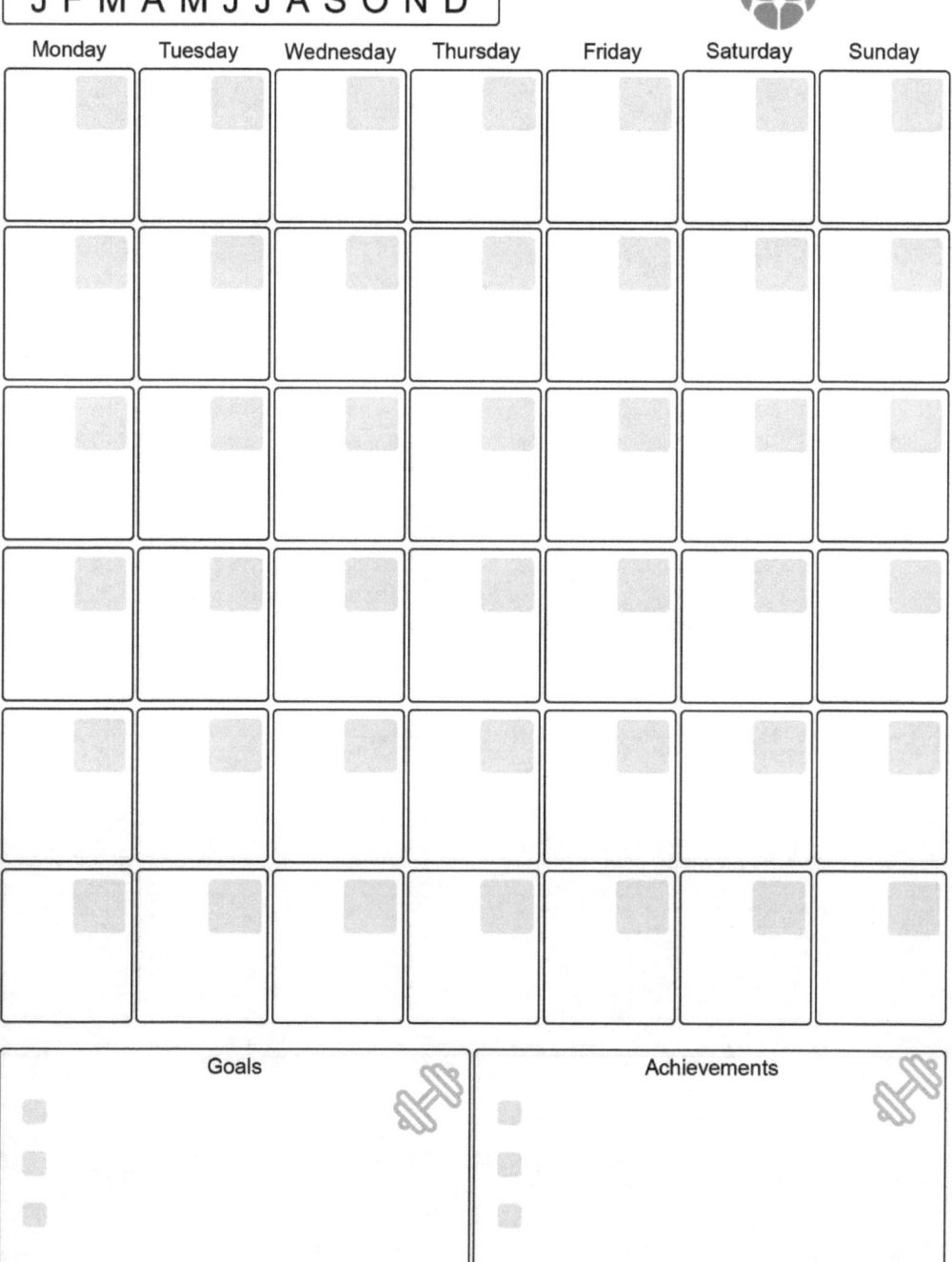

Fitness Calendar

Year:

J F M A M J J A S O N D

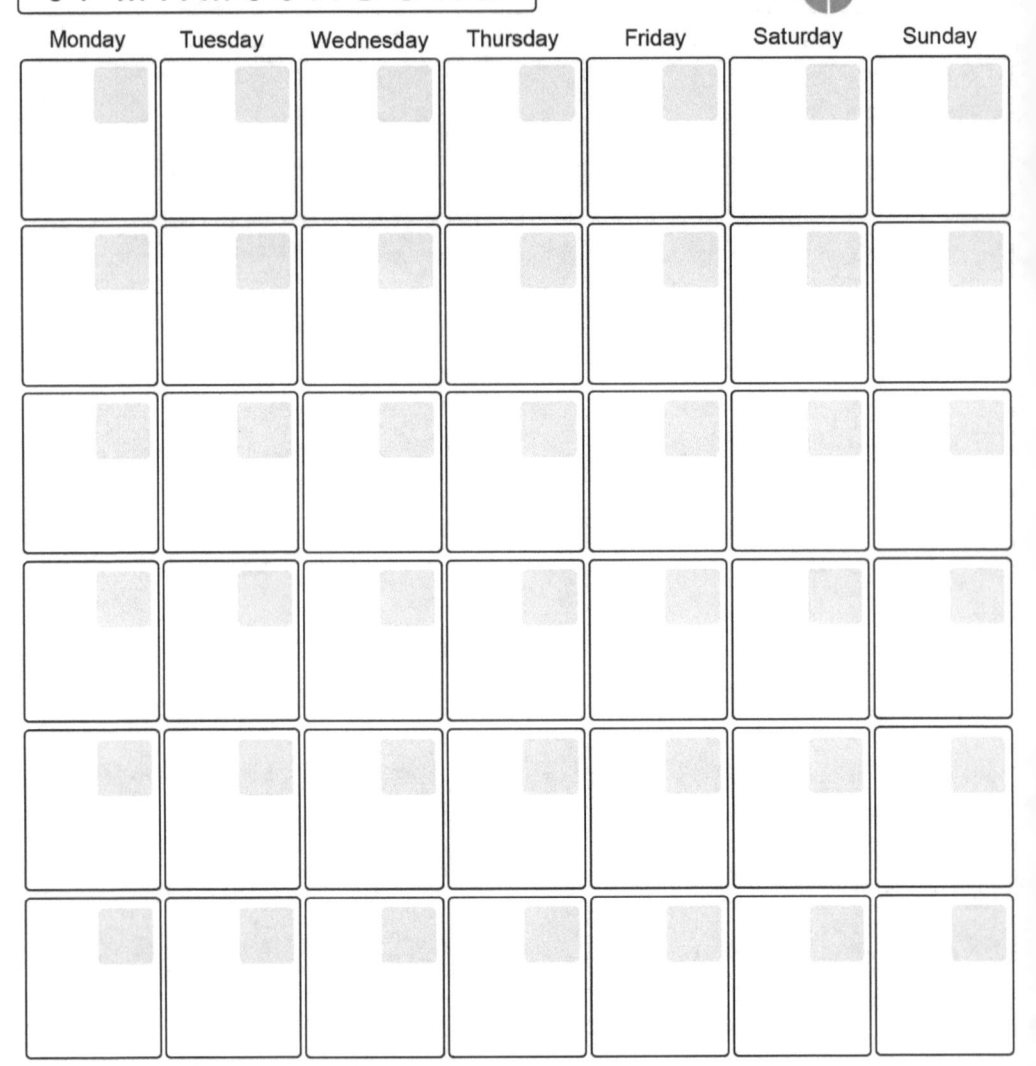

Monday	Tuesday	Wednesday	Thursday	Friday	Saturday	Sunday

Goals

Achievements